FIT TO LIFE

Balancing Physical, Mental, Emotional, and Spiritual Well-being.

ADELOWOKAN LIFTED

MAGCYART

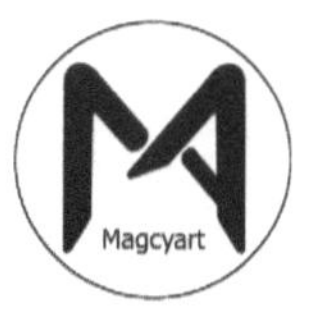

CONTENTS

INTRODUCTION

Welcome to "Fit to Life," a guide designed to help you navigate the complexities of modern living and find a sense of peace and fulfillment. This book delves into the emotional and mental challenges that many of us face, offering practical solutions and insights to help you achieve a balanced and harmonious life.

Purpose and Scope of the Book

The primary purpose of "Fit to Life" is to provide readers with tools and strategies to overcome worry, anxiety, and emotional turmoil. Through personal stories, practical advice, and reflective exercises, each chapter aims to guide you towards a state of inner peace and resilience. This book is not just a collection of theories but a heartfelt compilation of lived experiences and the wisdom gained from them.

Author's Motivation

The motivation behind "Fit to Life" is deeply rooted in a Judaic perspective, which emphasizes the importance of attachment and connection. In Judaism, the concept of d'vekut, or attachment, refers to a profound and sustaining connection to God, others, and oneself. It is believed that through these connections, one can achieve a sense of purpose, fulfillment, and emotional well-being.

In a broader sense, this perspective teaches that true peace and contentment come from maintaining healthy relationships and a strong sense of community. This attachment nurtures our soul, providing the strength to overcome life's challenges. "Fit to Life" incorporates this wisdom by encouraging readers to cultivate meaningful connections and a deep sense of attachment in their own lives.

In this book, you will explore how to:

- Develop self-awareness to understand the roots of your worries and emotional pain.

- Manage overthinking and find mental clarity.

- Cultivate inner peace and maintain emotional balance in daily life.

- Build and nurture supportive relationships that contribute to your overall well-being.

- Achieve emotional freedom and mental strength through the practice of meaningful attachment.

By integrating these concepts, "Fit to Life" aims to help you forge a path toward emotional freedom and mental strength, rooted in the timeless wisdom of attachment and connection. As you embark on this journey, may you find the peace and fulfillment that you seek.

CHAPTER 1: PHYSICAL FITNESS

Physical fitness is the foundation of a healthy and vibrant life. It encompasses various components that work together to ensure your body can perform daily activities efficiently and effectively. In this chapter, we will explore the definition and benefits of physical fitness, outline different types of exercise routines, discuss nutrition principles, and provide strategies for overcoming common obstacles. By the end of this chapter, you'll have a solid understanding of building and maintaining physical fitness in your life.

Definition and Benefits

Physical fitness is the ability to perform daily activities with vigor and without undue fatigue. It includes several components:

- Cardiovascular Endurance: The ability of your heart and lungs to supply oxygen during sustained physical activity. This component is crucial for activities like running, swimming, and cycling.

- Muscular Strength: The amount of force a muscle can produce in a single effort. Strength training exercises such as lifting weights or doing push-ups enhance this aspect.

- Flexibility: The range of motion available at a joint. Activities like yoga and stretching help maintain and improve flexibility.

- Body Composition: The ratio of fat to lean mass (muscles, bones, organs) in your body. Achieving a healthy body composition is often a result of regular physical activity and proper nutrition.

The benefits of physical fitness extend beyond the physical body:

- Improved Mental Health: Regular exercise can reduce symptoms of depression and anxiety, improve mood, and enhance cognitive function. It releases endorphins, which are chemicals in the brain that act as natural painkillers and mood elevators.

- Increased Energy Levels: Physical activity improves the efficiency of the cardiovascular system, which means more oxygen and nutrients are delivered to tissues, resulting in increased energy.

- Enhanced Overall Quality of Life: Being physically fit improves your ability to perform everyday tasks, reduces the risk of chronic diseases, and contributes to a longer, healthier life.

Exercise Routine

Types of Exercise: Cardio, Strength, Flexibility

To achieve a balanced physical fitness program, it's important to include different types of exercise:

- Cardiovascular Exercise: Activities such as running, brisk walking, swimming, and cycling increase heart rate and improve cardiovascular endurance. Aim for at least 150 minutes of moderate-intensity or 75 minutes of high-intensity cardio exercise per week.

- Strength Training: Exercises like weight lifting, resistance band workouts, and bodyweight exercises (e.g., squats, push-ups) build muscular strength. Include strength training exercises at least two days per week, targeting major muscle groups.

- Flexibility Exercises: Stretching, yoga, and pilates improve flexibility and reduce the risk of injury. Incorporate flexibility exercises into your routine on most days of the week.

Weekly Workout Plan

Creating a weekly workout plan ensures you cover all aspects of physical fitness. Here's an example:

- Monday: 30 minutes of cardio (e.g., running or cycling)

- Tuesday: Strength training (upper body)

- Wednesday* 30 minutes of cardio (e.g., swimming) + flexibility exercises (yoga)

- Thursday: Strength training (lower body)

- Friday: 30 minutes of cardio (e.g., brisk walking) + flexibility exercises (stretching)

- Saturday: Full-body strength training

- Sunday: Rest or light activity (e.g., walking, stretching)

Adjust this plan according to your fitness level and goals. The key is consistency and gradually increasing the intensity and duration of your workouts.

Nutrition

Basic Principles and Balanced Diet;

Nutrition plays a critical role in supporting physical fitness. Understanding the basic principles of a balanced diet helps you fuel your body properly:

- Macronutrients: Include carbohydrates, proteins, and fats in your diet. Carbohydrates provide energy, proteins build and repair tissues, and fats support cell function and hormone production.

- Micronutrients: Vitamins and minerals are essential for overall health. Ensure a varied diet that includes fruits, vegetables, lean proteins, whole grains, and healthy fats to meet your micronutrient needs.

- Portion Control: Be mindful of portion sizes to maintain a healthy weight. Use smaller plates, measure servings, and avoid eating directly from large containers.

Hydration Importance;

Staying hydrated is vital for physical performance and overall health. Water regulates body temperature, lubricates joints, and transports nutrients. Aim to drink at least 8-10 glasses of water per day, more if you are active or live in a hot climate. During exercise, drink water before, during, and after your workout to stay hydrated.

Overcoming Obstacles

Time Management

Finding time for exercise can be challenging, but it's essential to prioritize your fitness. Here are some tips:

- Schedule Workouts: Treat exercise like an important appointment. Schedule it into your calendar and stick to it.

- Break It Up: If you don't have time for a long workout, break it into shorter sessions throughout the day. Three 10-minute sessions are just as effective as one 30-minute session.

- Combine Activities: Integrate physical activity into your daily routine. Walk or bike to work, take the stairs, or do exercises while watching TV.

Handling Injuries

Injuries can disrupt your fitness routine, but they don't have to stop you completely:

- Prevent Injuries: Warm up before workouts, use proper form, and listen to your body.

- Manage Injuries: If you get injured, follow the R.I.C.E. method (Rest, Ice, Compression, Elevation) and consult a healthcare professional if necessary.

- Modify Workouts: Find alternative exercises that don't aggravate your injury. For example, if you have a lower-body injury, focus on upper-body exercises.

Staying Motivated

Maintaining motivation is key to long-term success in fitness:

- Set Goals: Set specific, measurable, achievable, relevant, and time-bound (SMART) goals to stay focused.

- Track Progress: Keep a fitness journal or use apps to track your workouts and progress.

- Find Support: Work out with a friend, join a fitness class, or find an online community for encouragement and accountability.

- Celebrate Successes: Reward yourself for reaching milestones, no matter how small. Celebrating your achievements keeps you motivated and committed.

By understanding the components and benefits of physical fitness, creating a balanced exercise routine, following proper nutrition guidelines, and overcoming common obstacles, you can build a strong foundation for a healthy and active life. Remember, consistency is key, and every step you take towards improving your physical fitness brings you closer to being "fit to life."

CHAPTER 2: MENTAL FITNESS

Mental fitness is essential for overall well-being, just as crucial as physical fitness. It involves maintaining a healthy mind that can handle stress, stay focused, and sustain emotional balance. In this chapter, we will explore the definition and importance of mental fitness, strategies for building resilience, ways to enhance cognitive function, and tips for maintaining mental health.

Understanding Mental Fitness;

Definition and Importance

Mental fitness refers to a state of well-being in which an individual realizes their abilities, can cope with the normal stresses of life, can work productively and fruitfully, and can contribute to their community. It involves:

- Emotional Stability: Being able to manage and express emotions appropriately.

- Psychological Resilience: The ability to recover quickly from difficulties.

- Cognitive Function: Efficient thinking processes, memory, and problem-solving skills.

The importance of mental fitness cannot be overstated. It affects how we think, feel, and act. It also helps determine how we handle stress, relate to others, and make choices. Mental fitness is vital at every stage of life, from childhood and adolescence through adulthood.

Building Resilience

Stress Management Techniques

Effective stress management is a cornerstone of mental fitness. Here are some techniques:

- Exercise: Physical activity reduces stress hormones and stimulates the production of endorphins, which are natural mood lifters.

- Deep Breathing: Techniques such as diaphragmatic breathing can activate the body's relaxation response, reducing stress.

- Time Management: Prioritizing tasks and breaking them into manageable steps can reduce feelings of overwhelm.

Sleep and Relaxation

Adequate sleep and relaxation are critical for mental fitness:

- Sleep Hygiene: Maintain a regular sleep schedule, create a restful environment, and avoid caffeine and electronics before bedtime to improve sleep quality.

- Relaxation Techniques: Practices such as progressive muscle relaxation, guided imagery, and listening to calming music can help relax the mind and body.

Mindfulness Practices

Mindfulness involves staying present and fully engaging with the current moment. Benefits include reduced stress, enhanced emotional regulation, and improved focus. Techniques include:

- Meditation: Daily meditation practice can increase mindfulness and reduce stress.

- Mindful Breathing: Focus on your breath to anchor yourself in the present moment.

- Mindful Activities: Engage in activities like walking, eating, or even cleaning with full attention to the experience.

Cognitive Function

Brain Exercises

Just like physical muscles, the brain benefits from regular exercise:

- Puzzles and Games: Activities like crosswords, Sudoku, and chess challenge the brain and improve cognitive function.

- Learning New Skills: Taking up new hobbies or learning new skills stimulates the brain.

- Memory Exercises: Techniques such as mnemonic devices and visualization can enhance memory.

Lifelong Learning

Continuous learning keeps the brain active and engaged:

- Reading: Regular reading expands knowledge and stimulates the mind.
- Courses and Workshops: Enroll in classes or attend workshops on topics of interest.
- Engaging Conversations: Discussing ideas and concepts with others can sharpen cognitive skills and expand perspectives.

Maintaining Mental Health

Recognizing Issues

Being aware of the signs and symptoms of mental health issues is crucial:

- Mood Changes: Persistent sadness, irritability, or anxiety.
- Behavioral Changes: Withdrawal from social activities, changes in eating or sleeping patterns.
- Cognitive Changes: Difficulty concentrating, remembering, or making decisions.

Seeking Help

If you recognize mental health issues, seeking help is essential:

- Professional Support: Therapists, counselors, and psychiatrists can provide diagnosis and treatment.
- Support Groups: Joining groups for specific conditions can

provide shared experiences and support.

- Self-Help Resources: Books, online courses, and apps can offer guidance and strategies for managing mental health.

Social Support

Strong social connections contribute significantly to mental fitness:

- Building Relationships: Cultivate relationships with family, friends, and colleagues.

- Community Involvement: Participate in community activities and volunteer work.

- Communicating: Open up about your feelings and experiences with trusted individuals.

By understanding the importance of mental fitness, building resilience, enhancing cognitive function, and maintaining overall mental health, you can achieve a balanced and fulfilling life. Mental fitness is an ongoing process that requires attention and effort, but the rewards are profound and long-lasting. Remember, taking care of your mind is just as important as taking care of your body. Stay committed to your mental fitness journey and embrace the positive changes it brings.

CHAPTER 3: EMOTIONAL FITNESS

Emotional fitness is a vital aspect of overall well-being, influencing how we navigate life's ups and downs. It involves understanding and managing emotions, building strong relationships, and practicing self-care. In this chapter, we will explore the definition and significance of emotional fitness, strategies for emotional resilience, the importance of relationships, and the role of self-care.

Understanding Emotional Fitness

Definition and Significance

Emotional fitness refers to the ability to understand, manage, and express emotions effectively. It encompasses emotional awareness, emotional regulation, and the ability to form healthy relationships. The significance of emotional fitness includes:

- Enhanced Well-Being: Emotionally fit individuals experience higher levels of happiness and life satisfaction.

- Improved Relationships: Emotional fitness fosters better communication, empathy, and stronger connections with others.

- Resilience: It provides the tools to cope with stress, adversity, and challenges in a healthy way.

Emotional Resilience

Coping Strategies

Developing effective coping strategies is essential for emotional resilience:

- Mindfulness and Meditation: Practicing mindfulness helps in staying present and reducing stress. Meditation can calm the mind and enhance emotional clarity.

- Physical Activity: Regular exercise releases endorphins, which can improve mood and reduce stress.

- Creative Outlets: Engaging in activities like art, music, or writing can be therapeutic and help process emotions.

Gratitude and Positivity

Cultivating gratitude and a positive outlook can significantly enhance emotional fitness:

- Gratitude Journaling: Writing down things you are grateful for each day can shift focus from negative to positive experiences.

- Positive Affirmations: Repeating positive affirmations can boost self-esteem and emotional strength.

- Surrounding Yourself with Positivity: Spend time with positive people and engage in uplifting activities.

Emotional Regulation

Managing emotions effectively is crucial for emotional resilience:

- Identifying Emotions: Recognize and name your emotions to understand them better.

- Healthy Expression: Express emotions in a healthy way, such as talking to someone you trust or engaging in creative activities.

- Relaxation Techniques: Practices such as deep breathing, progressive muscle relaxation, and visualization can help regulate intense emotions.

Relationships

Communication Skills

Effective communication is the foundation of healthy relationships:

- Active Listening: Truly listen to others without interrupting and respond thoughtfully.

- Clear Expression: Communicate your thoughts and feelings clearly and respectfully.

- Nonverbal Communication: Pay attention to body language, facial expressions, and tone of voice.

Building Healthy Relationships

Strong, healthy relationships are built on trust, respect, and mutual support:

- Trust and Honesty: Be honest and trustworthy in your

interactions.

- Support and Encouragement: Offer support and encouragement to others and seek it in return.

- Mutual Respect: Respect the boundaries and individuality of others.

Conflict Resolution

Effectively resolving conflicts is key to maintaining healthy relationships:

- Stay Calm: Approach conflicts with a calm and open mind.

- Understand Perspectives: Try to see the situation from the other person's perspective.

- Find Common Ground: Work together to find a mutually acceptable solution.

Self-Care

Importance of Routines

Establishing routines can provide stability and predictability:

- Daily Habits: Create daily routines that include time for self-care, relaxation, and activities you enjoy.

- Consistent Sleep Schedule: Maintain a regular sleep schedule to ensure adequate rest.

- Healthy Lifestyle: Incorporate a balanced diet, regular exercise, and sufficient hydration into your routine.

Activities for Well-Being

Engage in activities that promote well-being and relaxation:

- Hobbies and Interests: Pursue hobbies and interests that bring joy and fulfillment.

- Social Activities: Spend time with friends and loved ones to strengthen social connections.

- Relaxation Practices: Practice yoga, meditation, or other relaxation techniques to reduce stress.

Setting Boundaries

Setting and maintaining boundaries is essential for self-care and emotional fitness:

- Know Your Limits: Understand your limits and communicate them clearly to others.

- Say No When Needed: Don't be afraid to say no to requests or activities that overwhelm you.

- Prioritize Yourself: Make time for yourself and prioritize your own needs and well-being.

By understanding emotional fitness, building resilience, fostering healthy relationships, and practicing self-care, you can enhance your overall quality of life. Emotional fitness is a continuous journey of self-awareness, growth, and balance. Embrace this journey, and you will find greater emotional stability, stronger connections, and a more fulfilling life.

CHAPTER 4: SPIRITUAL FITNESS

Spiritual fitness is an often overlooked yet profoundly important aspect of overall well-being. It involves finding a sense of purpose, meaning, and connection beyond oneself. In this chapter, we will explore the definition and personal interpretation of spiritual fitness, discuss various spiritual practices, delve into discovering purpose and meaning, and provide strategies for daily integration of spiritual practices.

Understanding Spiritual Fitness

Definition and Personal Interpretation

Spiritual fitness refers to the state of being connected to something greater than oneself, which can provide a sense of purpose and meaning in life. It is a deeply personal aspect of well-being that varies greatly from person to person. It can include religious beliefs, a connection to nature, or a commitment to certain values and principles. The significance of spiritual fitness includes:

- Inner Peace: A deep sense of calm and contentment.

- Purpose and Direction: Clear understanding of one's values and goals.

- Connection: Feeling connected to others and the world around you.

Spiritual Practices

Meditation and Mindfulness

Meditation and mindfulness are powerful practices that enhance spiritual fitness:

- Meditation: This practice involves focusing the mind and eliminating distractions to achieve a state of deep peace and heightened awareness. Techniques can include breath-focused meditation, mantra meditation, and visualization.

- Mindfulness: Being fully present in the moment, mindfulness can help you appreciate the beauty of everyday experiences and reduce stress.

Prayer and Reflection

For many, prayer and reflection are central to spiritual fitness:

- Prayer: A form of communication with a higher power, prayer can offer comfort, guidance, and a sense of connection. It can be structured or spontaneous, silent or spoken.

- Reflection: Regular periods of reflection, such as journaling or quiet contemplation, can help you process experiences and gain insight into your spiritual journey.

Connecting with Nature

Nature can be a profound source of spiritual inspiration and renewal:

- Nature Walks: Spending time in natural settings, such as forests, parks, or by the sea, can foster a sense of peace and connectedness.

- Gardening: Engaging with the earth and nurturing plant life can be a meditative and spiritually enriching activity.

- Mindful Observation: Simply observing the natural world—the movement of clouds, the rustling of leaves, the flow of water—can be deeply calming and spiritually uplifting.

Purpose and Meaning

Discovering Values and Beliefs

Understanding your core values and beliefs is essential for spiritual fitness:

- Self-Reflection: Take time to reflect on what truly matters to you. What principles guide your actions? What gives your life meaning?

- Exploration: Read books, attend lectures, and engage in discussions to explore different spiritual perspectives and philosophies.

- Values Assessment: Identify your core values and how they align with your daily actions and decisions.

Setting Goals

Setting meaningful goals that align with your values can enhance your sense of purpose:

- Short-Term Goals: Establish achievable short-term goals that reflect your values and contribute to your overall purpose.

- Long-Term Goals: Define long-term aspirations that give you a sense of direction and motivation.

- Regular Review: Periodically review and adjust your goals to ensure they remain aligned with your evolving values and beliefs.

Living Purposefully

Living a purposeful life involves aligning your actions with your values and goals:

- Intentional Living: Make conscious choices that reflect your values and contribute to your long-term goals.

- Service to Others: Engage in activities that benefit others, whether through volunteer work, acts of kindness, or professional endeavors that align with your values.

- Mindful Presence: Strive to be fully present and engaged in each moment, recognizing the significance of your actions and interactions.

Daily Integration

Daily Spiritual Practices

Incorporating spiritual practices into your daily routine can foster ongoing spiritual growth:

- Morning Rituals: Start your day with practices such as meditation, prayer, or reading inspirational texts.

- Evening Reflection: End your day with reflection or gratitude journaling to review the day's experiences and express thanks.

- Mindfulness Breaks: Take short breaks throughout the day to practice mindfulness and reconnect with your spiritual self.

Balancing Life Aspects

Balancing various aspects of your life is essential for holistic spiritual fitness:

- Work-Life Balance: Ensure that your professional life aligns with your values and allows time for personal and spiritual activities.

- Self-Care: Prioritize self-care practices that nurture your body, mind, and spirit.

- Relationships: Foster healthy relationships that support your spiritual growth and provide mutual support.

Community Involvement

Engaging with a community can enhance your sense of connection and purpose:

- Join Groups: Participate in spiritual or religious groups, clubs, or organizations that align with your values and beliefs.

- Volunteer: Offer your time and skills to causes and organizations that resonate with your sense of purpose.

- Build Connections: Develop meaningful relationships with others who share your spiritual outlook and values.

By understanding spiritual fitness, engaging in meaningful

practices, discovering your purpose, and integrating these elements into daily life, you can achieve a deeper sense of fulfillment and well-being. Spiritual fitness is a journey of continuous exploration and growth, offering profound rewards along the way. Embrace this journey, and you will find greater peace, purpose, and connection in your life.

CHAPTER 5: BRINGING IT ALL TOGETHER

As we come to the end of our journey through "Fit to Life," it's important to reflect on the holistic approach we've explored to achieve overall well-being. This chapter will recap the key points from each aspect of fitness—physical, mental, emotional, and spiritual—while offering encouragement for ongoing self-improvement and some final motivational thoughts.

Recap of Key Points

Chapter 1: Physical Fitness

- Definition and Benefits: Physical fitness involves the ability to perform daily activities with vigor and without undue fatigue, encompassing cardiovascular endurance, muscular strength, flexibility, and body composition. Benefits include improved mental health, increased energy levels, and enhanced quality of life.

- Exercise Routine: A balanced exercise routine should include cardio, strength training, and flexibility exercises. A weekly workout plan helps maintain consistency and progress.

- Nutrition: Proper nutrition involves a balanced diet rich in essential nutrients and adequate hydration, which are crucial for optimal physical performance and health.

- Overcoming Obstacles: Effective time management, injury prevention, and sustained motivation are key to overcoming challenges in maintaining physical fitness.

Chapter 2: Mental Fitness

- Understanding Mental Fitness: Mental fitness refers to maintaining a state of well-being and the ability to manage stress, enhance cognitive function, and maintain a positive mental state.

- Building Resilience: Techniques such as stress management, adequate sleep, relaxation, and mindfulness practices are essential for building mental resilience.

- Cognitive Function: Brain exercises and lifelong learning are important for maintaining and improving cognitive abilities.

- Maintaining Mental Health: Recognizing mental health issues, seeking help when needed, and fostering social support are crucial for ongoing mental well-being.

Chapter 3: Emotional Fitness

- Understanding Emotional Fitness: Emotional fitness involves understanding and managing emotions, building strong relationships, and practicing self-care.

- Emotional Resilience: Coping strategies, gratitude, positivity, and emotional regulation are vital for emotional stability.

- Relationships: Effective communication, healthy relationships, and conflict resolution skills are key components of emotional fitness.

- Self-Care: Establishing routines, engaging in activities that promote well-being, and setting boundaries are essential for maintaining emotional health.

Chapter 4: Spiritual Fitness

- Understanding Spiritual Fitness: Spiritual fitness is about finding a sense of purpose, meaning, and connection beyond oneself, which can be deeply personal and varied.

- Spiritual Practices: Practices such as meditation, mindfulness, prayer, reflection, and connecting with nature can enhance spiritual well-being.

- Purpose and Meaning: Discovering personal values and beliefs, setting meaningful goals, and living purposefully contribute to a fulfilling spiritual life.

- Daily Integration: Incorporating daily spiritual practices, balancing life aspects, and engaging with a community can help sustain spiritual fitness.

Encouragement for Ongoing Self-Improvement

Achieving fitness in all these areas is not a one-time effort but a continuous journey. Here are some tips to keep you motivated and committed to ongoing self-improvement:

- Set Realistic Goals: Start with small, achievable goals and gradually increase the challenges as you progress.

- Stay Consistent: Consistency is key. Make your fitness routines a regular part of your daily life.

- Seek Support: Surround yourself with supportive friends, family, or communities that share your commitment to well-being.

- Reflect Regularly: Take time to reflect on your progress, celebrate your achievements, and identify areas for improvement.

- Stay Positive: Keep a positive mindset and remember that setbacks are part of the journey. Use them as learning opportunities.

Final Motivational Thoughts

As you continue your journey towards a balanced and fulfilling life, remember that each step you take brings you closer to your goals. Embrace the process and be patient with yourself. Here are some final thoughts to keep you inspired:

- Believe in Yourself: You have the power to create the life you want. Trust in your abilities and stay committed to your path.

- Embrace Change: Change is inevitable and can be a powerful catalyst for growth. Be open to new experiences and learning opportunities.

- Find Joy in the Journey: Focus not just on the destination but on enjoying the journey itself. Each moment offers a chance to grow and improve.

- Live Authentically: Stay true to your values and beliefs. Authenticity leads to genuine happiness and fulfillment.

By integrating the principles of physical, mental, emotional, and spiritual fitness into your daily life, you can achieve a well-rounded, healthy, and fulfilling life. Keep moving forward, stay motivated, and remember that you are "Fit to Life."

Thank you for joining me on this journey. Here's to your health, happiness, and continued growth!

ABOUT THE AUTHOR

Adelowokan Lifted

The author of "Fit to Life" has navigated a life filled with worries and emotional challenges. Overthinking became a constant companion, affecting even the smallest aspects of daily life. Despite these struggles, the author discovered effective ways to overcome these hurdles and find peace of mind.

Drawing from personal experiences, each chapter of "Fit to Life" delves into the transformative journey from a life overwhelmed by anxiety to one of balance and tranquility. The book is a testament to the belief that achieving a "Fit to Life" requires nurturing mental well-being and cultivating inner peace. Through these pages, the author shares valuable insights and practical strategies that have made a significant difference in their life, offering readers a path to their own emotional resilience and harmony.

www.ingramcontent.com/pod-product-compliance
Lightning Source LLC
Chambersburg PA
CBHW051406250726
48656CB00006B/2287

* 9 7 9 8 3 2 8 7 0 5 6 1 5 *